NO

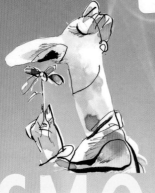
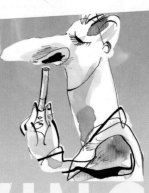

SMOKING

NO
SMOKING

© Fitway Publishing, 2004.
Original editions in French, English, Spanish, Italian

All rights reserved, including partial or complete translation,
adaptation and reproduction rights,
in any form and for any purpose

Translation by Translate-A-Book, Oxford

Design and creation: GRAPH'M

ISBN: 2-7528-0088-6
Publisher code: T00088

Copyright registration: 2004 September
Printed in Singapore by Tien Wah Press

www.fitwaypublishing.com

Fitway Publishing
12, avenue d'Italie – 75627 Paris cedex 13

NO
SMOKING

pierre doncieux
illustrations jean-pierre cagnat

foreword dr vera luiza da costa e silva,
WHO's noncommunicable diseases and mental health

CON

TENTS

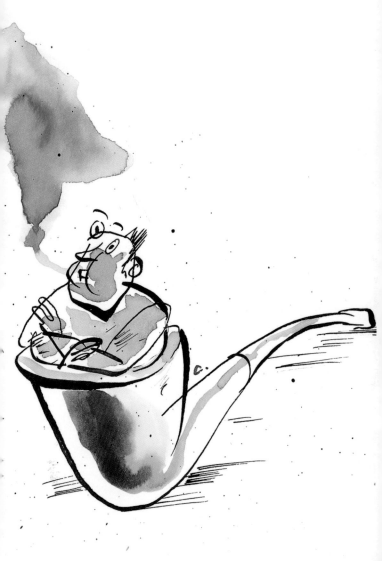

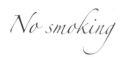

No smoking

Tobacco is the only legally available product that, when consumed as indicated by the manufacturer, kills half of its regular users. There are 1.3 billion smokers worldwide, one of whom dies from a tobacco-related disease every 6.5 seconds.

Around three-quarters of those who use tobacco would like to quit, but nicotine is a highly addictive substance. Helpful environments to support smokers in their efforts to quit are essential. Effective measures that can help include bans on tobacco advertising and smoking in public places, increased tobacco prices, taxes and information campaigns. The WHO Framework Convention on Tobacco Control, adopted by WHO Member States in May 2003, sets out minimum standards for these and other measures to help people stop using tobacco and to treat tobacco dependence.

No smoking

This book shows how good medical advice and sometimes treatment is necessary to beat the addiction to tobacco, and it emphasises the importance of support and encouragement from friends and family once tobacco users have taken the decision to quit.
Finally, it stresses the immense short- and long-term benefits of giving up tobacco, and the satisfaction of overcoming a life-threatening addiction.

I hope this book will sustain those who have decided to quit and encourage other tobacco users to do likewise.

Dr Vera Luiza da Costa e Silva, MD, PhD
Director, Tobacco Free Initiative (TFI)
WHO's Noncommunicable Diseases and Mental Health

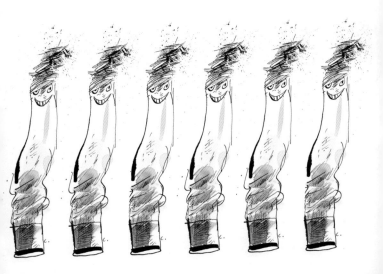

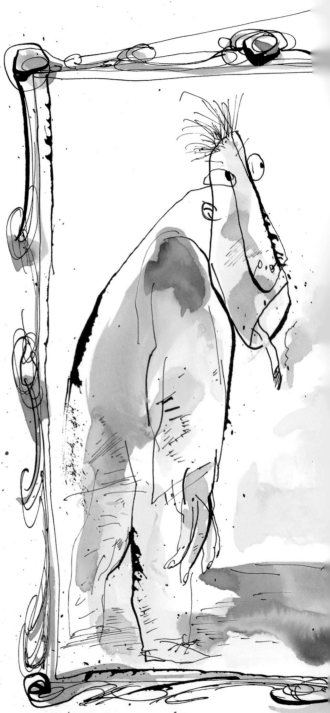

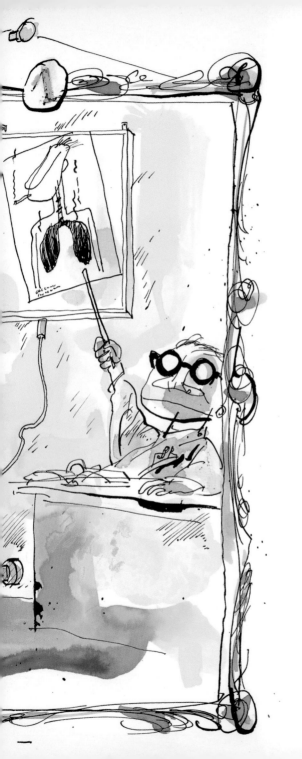

Why I'm stopping

I'm stopping smoking this morning and, to have any
chance of success, I shall have to turn everything upside
down. For example, no more breaks for coffee and
newspaper after dropping the eldest off at school: the
temptation would be too great. I've finished, had it.
I feel like a prisoner. I'm stopping in order to live better.
Among other things, to avoid that moment of recoil
before kissing my wife and children when I get home
in the evening, having 'had a drag' on my scooter.
The crunch came the day I realised that even a smoker's
breath could harm his family. The idea gradually took
hold. Mind you, this isn't my first attempt. I managed

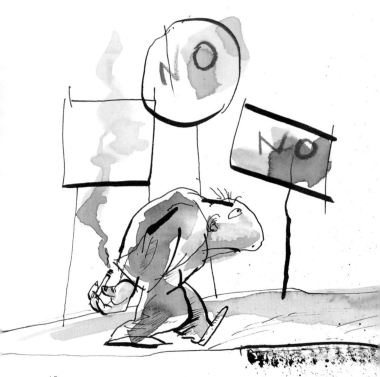

No smoking

three months the first time and twice that long at
the second attempt. That was five and ten years ago.
Both times it was a failure. To make sure it goes well
this time, I have taken advice. Indispensable, say former
smokers. Doctor G., our family practitioner, treated me
just like a real patient. The consultation lasted three-
quarters of an hour. Forty-five minutes during which
he described the difficulties produced by this decision.
He warned me it would be physically and psychologically
difficult. The doctor prescribed patches, the strongest,

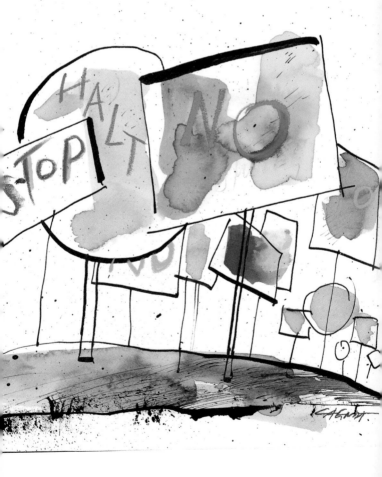

No smoking

since science views me as a person in danger. For twenty years I have inhaled the smoke of twenty to thirty strong Virginians every day. I am stopping because I want to be in love with life, not with a cigarette. I do not want to shorten it for the sake of a £2.67 fix. **From now on the watchword is 'hold on'.**

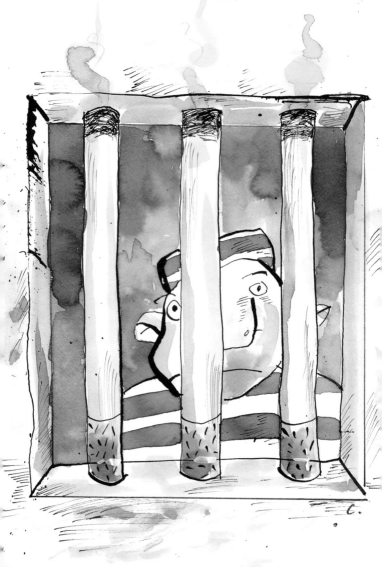

72 hours later: still no regrets, but I can't get it out of my head!

From time to time I try to remember. I inhale 'blanks'.
I imagine the smoke running over me. That delightful
'warm' feeling on the tongue, then, if the inhalation is a
long one, a slight feeling of suffocation as it passes down
the windpipe. The smoke continues on its way down to
hell, before returning. Complete exhalation, preferably
through the nose: I used to love exhaling this way. With
the calm rhythm of breathing, with nonchalance, I used
to take pleasure in allowing the smoke to come out of
my mouth while talking. Or whistling. Or blowing …
I expected to feel the need to keep my hands busy.
Now it's my mouth that needs something. This marathon
starts off at a sprint. I have to try, in the short term,
to forget about the cigarettes I lit every half-hour as
a smoker. Especially the best ones: the first smoke in
the morning, on the landing as soon as I came out of
the door, the cigarettes smoked 'after' — after lunch
and dinner, that is.

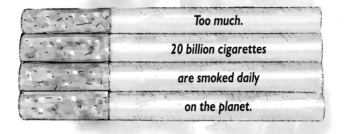

Too much.

20 billion cigarettes

are smoked daily

on the planet.

But the most difficult times are not the times I usually smoked. I can reason with myself as these approach. Worse are the unexpected sneak nicotine attacks, about which my patch and my brain can do nothing. An irresistible desire to smoke crops up when I am on the telephone, in a meeting, or having a conversation in the street. I get these attacks even when I emerge from the shower following an energetic game of tennis. These occurrences make me feel sad. But not aggressive, not yet. They last for ten minutes or so. I don't (yet) know how or with what I can subdue them. I grit my teeth. At dinner with friends the night before last we finished with dessert and coffee; a smoke, surely, comes next. I gave myself a last glass of red wine … while quietly inhaling curls of my neighbours' smoke. For the first time I was a victim of passive smoking. **What real luck!**

No smoking

Very dangerous. Tobacco is responsible for 5 per cent of world mortality; 10 per cent of that in France; 20 per cent in Great Britain and the United States.

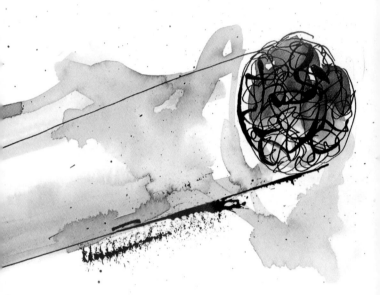

Abstaining. If one does not smoke for 14–16 hours, nearly all the nicotine in the body disappears.

One week later, watching for the smallest triumph over desire

Six days later, how's it going? So-so. First lesson: it is much easier to control one's dark desires at the weekend than it is during the week. Since Monday the days have been desperately long, even if they were full. The hours pass without interruption, without breathing. On Monday and Tuesday I had absolutely no wish to work. I didn't want anything else, either. A void. It is as though a quitting smoker puts all his energy into his objective, and tends to neglect everything else. I try to achieve a normal level of activity without my preoccupation showing. At least I hope it doesn't. I would like stopping to be a non-event, a nothing, the miserable ash of nothing at all. But I can't manage it. My mind tries to make up for my body's demands. I look for rewards, or for revenge for having made this decision. I have not

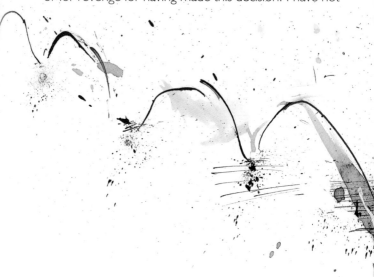

No smoking

yet dived into a shop to buy a bar of chocolate or three
Mars bars and scoff them in a few seconds. But I know
it will happen at any moment. It is beginning to show
at the table. The essential thing is still not to smoke.
Yesterday, the reason for holding out was financial.
A box of patches cost me £63 for fourteen days of
treatment, the rough equivalent of two weeks' tobacco
consumption. Clearly there's no big risk involved. At least
I ought to finish this box. Seen this way, it is already a
small triumph over desire. The game right now consists
of finding a good reason to hang on whenever there's
an urge to cave in, and to get through to the evening and
say: well done, for today. **Tomorrow, the struggle
continues.**

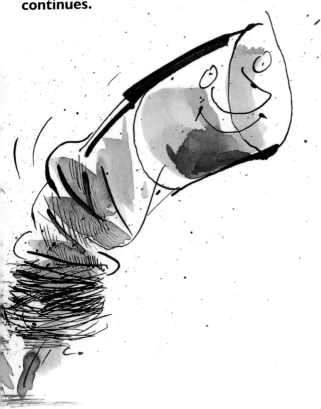

An ex-smoker is a twenty-first-century adventurer

Let's start with some thanks. This project has prompted numerous friendly, encouraging reactions. Not just from friends but from acquaintances too, sending e-mails or phoning to encourage yours truly. That's not to mention the members of my family who, again last night, unendingly praised my complexion and my calm demeanour, even if quitting has tended to make things

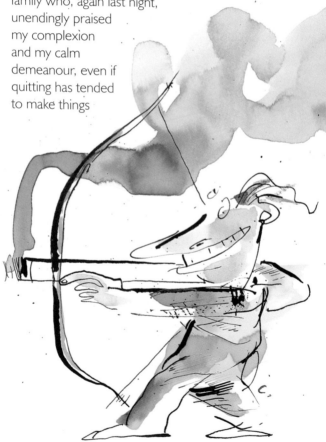

difficult when it comes to sleeping. From my (soon to be clean) heart, all thanks. It is a real support. Please carry on. I won't deny that sometimes I feel that these compliments are slightly 'forced'. Designed to comfort when I feel my motivation yielding. It happens. But it is not important. Those kind words reinforce the idea that stopping smoking is one of the great adventures of our century. Yes, let's not mince words. Like a sportsman

who trains physically, plans his tactics and psychologically conditions himself to win, the smoker uses the same weapons to (try to) reach his goals … and win.

Our civilisation has produced adventurers of all kinds, climbing the Himalayas, crossing the oceans, and so on. It has also invented nicotine adventurers. I am one of these. In this 'sport', the best go from three packets a day, or more, to nothing. I am a lightweight: I'm starting from thirty a day. The coach is my doctor, he is my carer. Victory is never total. **The road is beset with pitfalls.**

375 hours later, I'm already feeling much better, I think

Over two weeks, 360 hours. Come on! Every day without tobacco is still counted as a victory. There's no respite in the fight. You have to monitor yourself, concentrate, and motivate yourself continuously. But quitting is beginning to have some encouraging effects. For example: the feeling of great tiredness on the morning after an evening's drinking has become a bad memory. I'm all ready to go as soon as I have my coffee; in my case this is a real achievement. No more furry mouth first thing. That's good too. The rings round my eyes seem less obvious. 'Your skin is ten times nicer, and you smell a lot nicer, even your hair', comments my wife. Fancy that, she has never mentioned the smell of my hair before. At dinner my eldest confirms it. More than anything else, I see my family making an effort when the pressure mounts. Indeed, the smoker in withdrawal soon becomes irritable, unfair, and abusive – but not for long. That's good news (for the family).

Automatism. The rhythm of cigarette smoking is determined by changes in the level of nicotine in the blood, directed by the part of the brain that also automatically governs the levels of oxygen and glucose, and body temperature.

No smoking

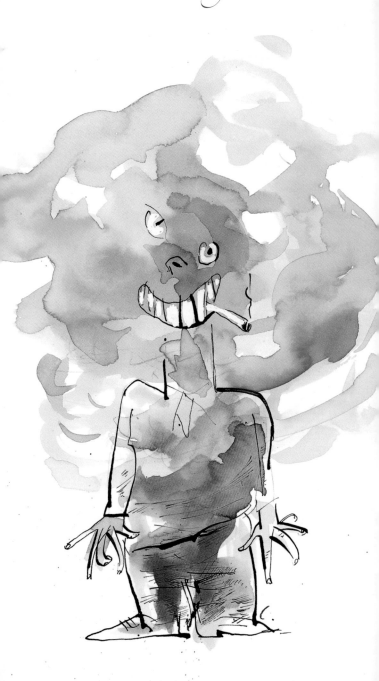

No smoking

There is also a real change of scene as regards my sense of smell. The fragrance of cigarettes still attracts me. I seek it out. But there are the smells of life too. This week at the office I detected one that was nauseating. I spent quite a while trying to find the source. Could it be so-and-so neglecting himself? I suspected my colleagues; even my partner. I can now identify smells that I had stopped recognising. Some are disturbing; others bring back pleasant memories, such as the smell of freshly-cut grass, a spring flower, or the complex oil-petrol blend of a two-stroke moped. Foods, too, have a different taste. There has been some effect on my weight, but I begin to tell myself that the sum of the advantages of a life without tobacco justifies the effort. Although a puff of smoke, deliciously pervading the mouth, invading the windpipe, descending to the lungs, then returning lazily to exit via the nostrils, is still classified as a pleasure. **You can't change that in a fortnight.**

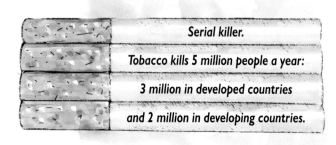

Serial killer.

Tobacco kills 5 million people a year:

3 million in developed countries

and 2 million in developing countries.

No smoking

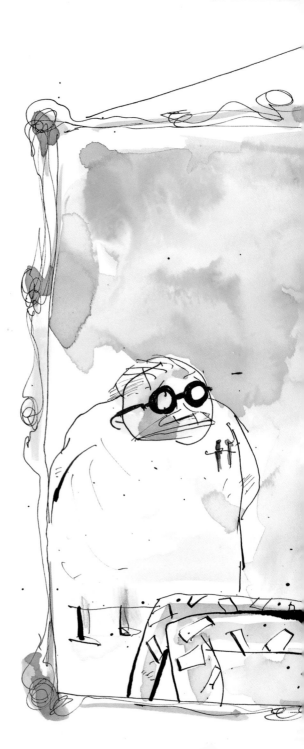

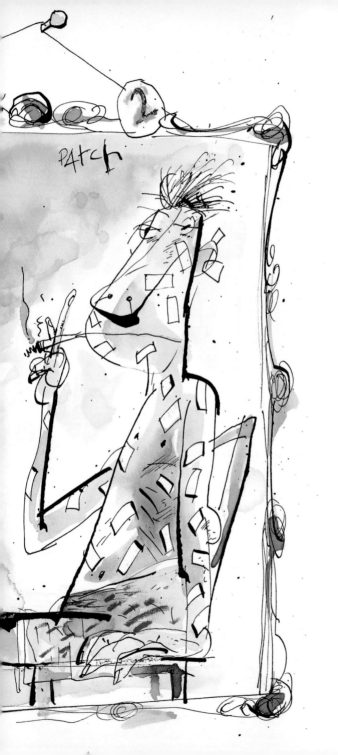

420 unsmoked cigarettes: it wears you down, though

One packet a day for three weeks, that makes 420 cigarettes, or about £57. Just about the price of the first box of patches. I had sworn to hold on for at least this length of time. It's a case of recovering the 'investment'. But it shouldn't be believed that cutting out tobacco automatically produces savings. Other sources of pleasure are needed: there are the sales, and the £38 invested in presents. Besides, I'm already thinking about the next one.

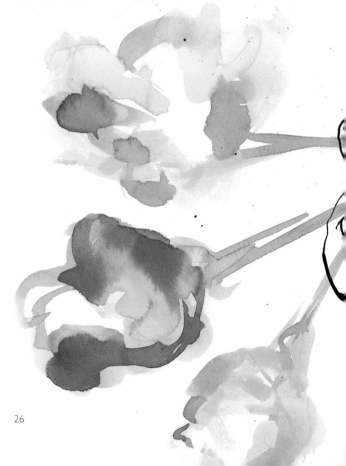

No smoking

I have eight patches left. I'll finish this box … then I'll go and buy another, at a lower dosage. I'm not counting on lasting that long, even if I do have the feeling of beginning a new, delicate phase. Stopping is in fact becoming a non-event. It is becoming ordinary. By now my family class me as a non-smoker, whereas sometimes desire tortures me terribly, all the more so when I have

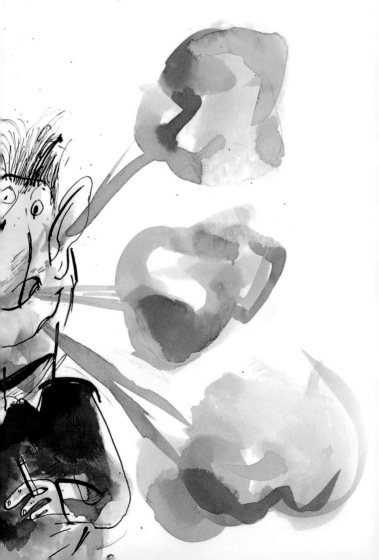

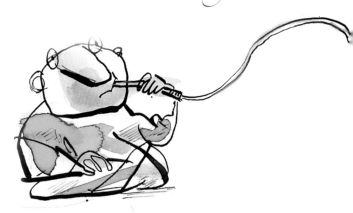

forgotten to put on the famous patch. That happened the day before yesterday. Despite everything I decided to do without it, just to see. I suffered in silence. The withdrawal symptoms were suddenly much stronger. I found it difficult to concentrate, I felt irritable and had no wish to work.

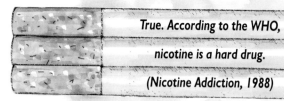

True. According to the WHO,

nicotine is a hard drug.

(Nicotine Addiction, 1988)

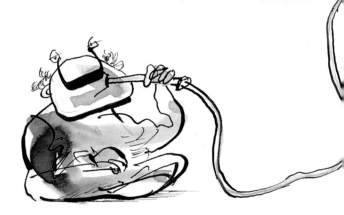

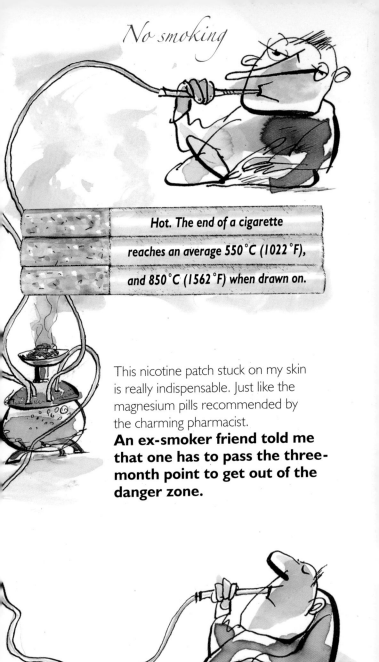

Hot. The end of a cigarette reaches an average 550°C (1022°F), and 850°C (1562°F) when drawn on.

This nicotine patch stuck on my skin is really indispensable. Just like the magnesium pills recommended by the charming pharmacist. **An ex-smoker friend told me that one has to pass the three-month point to get out of the danger zone.**

No smoking

My husband, the hero

While Pierre is very anxious not to think about tobacco, I, Sophie, his wife, will bring you up to date about my ex-smoker. We had planned to go away as a family for a few days at the end of the first month after he quit, on advice from a doctor friend of mine. And here we are in the country. We are on holiday, yet I can't remember ever having seen my husband so active, even agitated, engaged in cutting the grass, trimming the hedges, running after all sorts of balls (golf, tennis) and balloons. But, as my three well-meaning sisters-in-law would say, for the moment he's not running after a blonde. I have the impression he's tiring himself out to avoid thinking about cigarettes too much.

Another considerable change is that he doesn't know what to do with his hands, so he devours things, hovers about the kitchen, offers to do the shopping, swallows litres of Coca Cola and takes me in his arms a lot more than usual. I am really grateful for this incredible change. He is the hero of the moment. Out of love, he is accomplishing something for us. The rings round his eyes and his ashen complexion have almost disappeared, and he smells good: I spend my time sniffing at his hair, it's lovely! Nonetheless, I must say I have to watch myself over his temper. He throws tantrums for the stupidest reasons: but we stay calm. The family watchword for the summer is 'glide'. We have to glide over his sudden fits of temper, his occasional inappropriate remarks … glide, glide. Put on a serene smile and wipe the slate clean. He needs to be surrounded, congratulated and encouraged. **This is the way we, his family, contribute to the war effort.**

No smoking

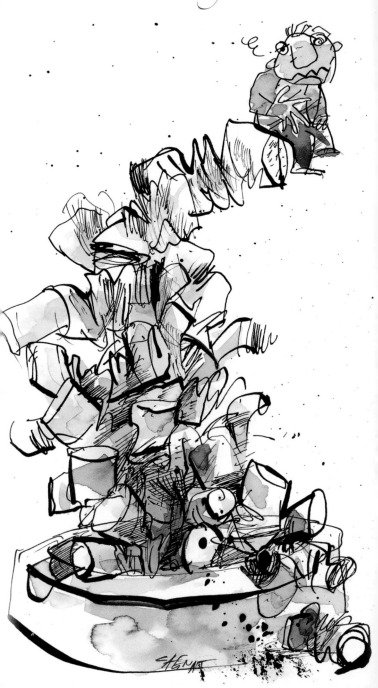

What makes me hold on? My nose!

Fifty days on and 1,500 cigarettes saved. Good. But it's nothing: according to the Marie Curie Institute in Paris, well-known for its research on tobacco, a hundred times as much time, just over 5,400 days (fifteen years!) is needed before my cells return to normal. This at least is a long-term objective, which should not mar the first symbolic stage. My own fiftieth anniversary …

This promptly provokes a thought: the life of an ex-smoker needs careful re-evaluation.

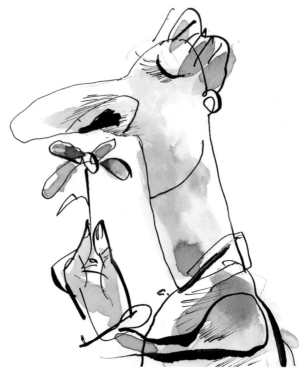

No smoking

The cigarette, that faithful year-long companion during
times of stress, and the one I'm trying to give up, for
good or bad, this cigarette becomes the object of all
desire during moments of relaxation, at the weekend and
on holiday. It used to be an intimate part of relaxation.
It embodied pleasure. From now on I have to learn to
enjoy myself without it. I have to mourn a second time.
My mind had actually removed the cigarette from its
'decompression valve for immoderate use' category;
now it also has to be removed from the 'pleasure'
category. Ah, a long puff at dusk before a glass of beer,
or before a port at the end of an excessively long dinner!
The variants are many and delightful to live through.
I look at smokers more than before. I watch them

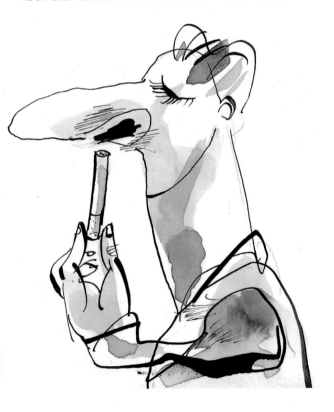

inhale and exhale. I open their cigarette packets, just to smell them. People around me become uneasy. The entire world holds its breath. I breathe in, lingering over the filters. Oh, it's so good! I rediscover the smell of packets stolen in my youth, smoked in no time, chain-smoked. Exactly the same smell. Olfactory memory is an increasingly real concept. Fortunately this ballad of smells is about much more than the filters. Hay or cut grass, flowers, trees, cooking and suntan oil also take me back to my childhood, bringing pleasant feelings, occasionally making me shudder. Smells act like an album of photos passing before my eyes. I'm holding on by means of my nose. Were it not for that, I would never make it. Smoking brings an illusion of pleasure. In reality, nicotine cuts us off from the 'real' world, from what one can smell. If smoking gradually made one blind instead of affecting the sense of smell, there would be many fewer smokers on this earth!
And stopping would be child's play.

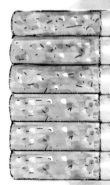

Dump. You can find everything

in cigarettes, including cocoa.

Cocoa contains theobromine which

dilates the bronchi and allows quicker

absorption of nicotine, thus allowing it

to reach the brain faster.

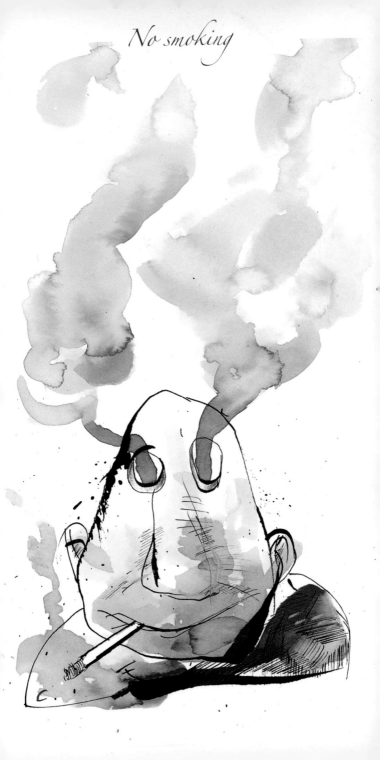

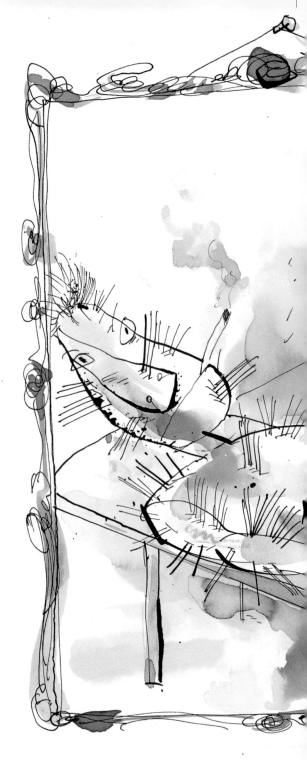

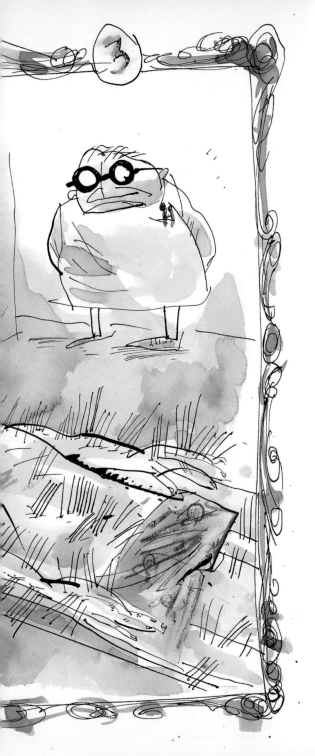

No smoking

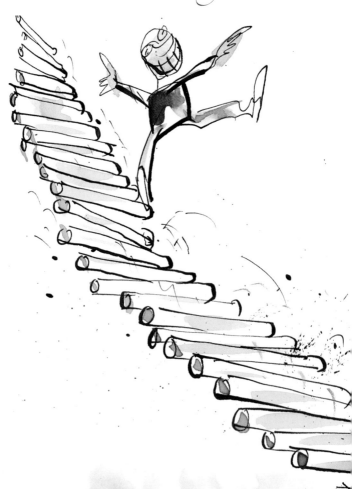

The risk of cancer of the colon is multiplied by 1.9 in those who smoke between 1 and 20 packets of cigarettes per year, and by 3.9 in those who smoke more than 20 packets.

Two months without smoking, but I'm not sleeping

The ex-smoker will confirm that, as the weeks go by, this pursuit makes one slightly paranoid. Conversation soon turns to the quitter's worries. Yours truly, for example, on meeting an old friend very familiar with health matters:

'Splendid! How did you do it? Patches, sedatives, both, nothing?'

'Patches for a month, then nothing more. It was my doctor's advice. They're really effective.'

'Well done. Not feeling nervous? Not putting on weight at all?'

'Nervous? Well, I don't know. I don't think so. My little family doesn't give me the impression of being terrorised and I don't yell at my wife any more. Weight? Not too much yet. I have put on 2 kilos (4.4 lb), at present. On the other hand, I'm sleeping really badly.'

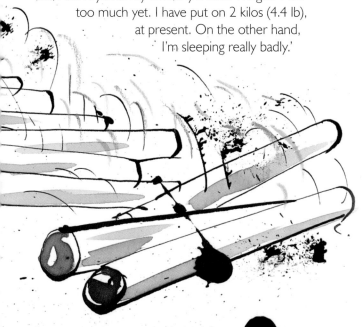

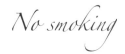

No smoking

'Oh really? Have you taken anything to help you?'

'No, not for the moment.'

'You should. Do you find it hard to get to sleep, or do you have insomnia?'

'Both. I wake up regularly every night towards four o'clock. Sometimes I don't fall asleep again. Or I wake at all hours and in the end I get up at dawn. It's very unpleasant and exhausting. I'm worn out all day. And I find it hard to get to sleep as well!'

'Yes. Do you feel depressed?'

'No, not at all, why?'

'Because this type of insomnia is typical of people who are slightly depressed. Are you sure that cutting out cigarettes isn't getting on your nerves?'

'It is a bit, certainly. I imagine you can't go from nearly two packets a day to no cigarettes without some collateral damage. Having said that, I don't feel sad, despondent or inactive during the day.'

'You should take some St John's Wort. It's a plant recognised as being effective in treating depressive states, anxiety and nervous agitation. Try it, you'll find you sleep better. And then you should go back and see your doctor.'

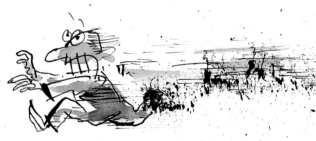

No smoking

'All right. Where can I find some St John's Wort? Do I collect it in the countryside?'

'Dummy, it's sold in capsules in any pharmacy.'

Two hours later, here I am asking my pharmacist for a box of St John's Wort.

'Something wrong?' he asks.

'No, everything's fine. I've just stopped smoking.'

'Obviously … now cheer up.'

That night I slept like a baby, right through.

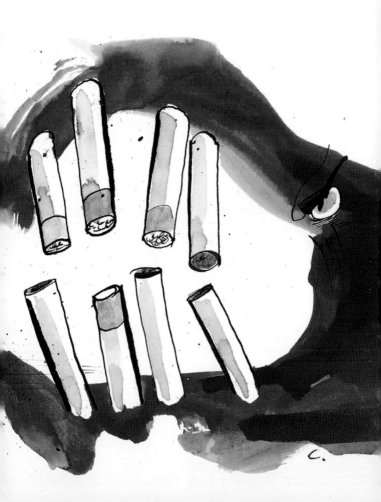

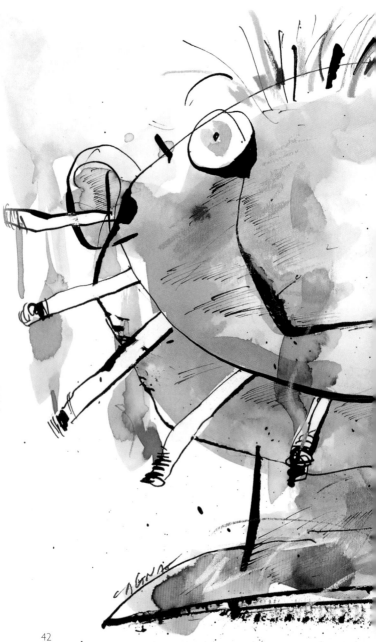

No smoking

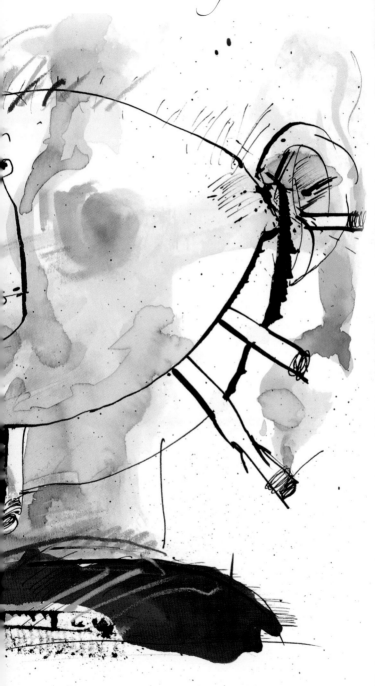

No smoking

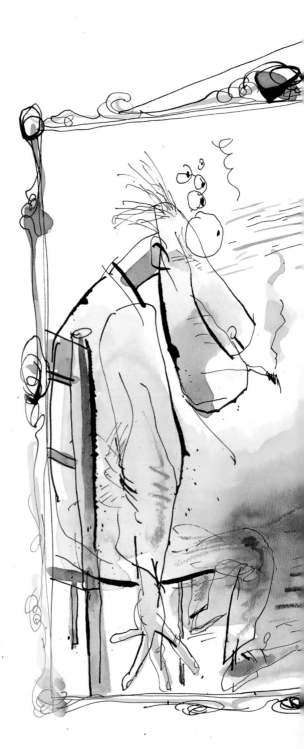

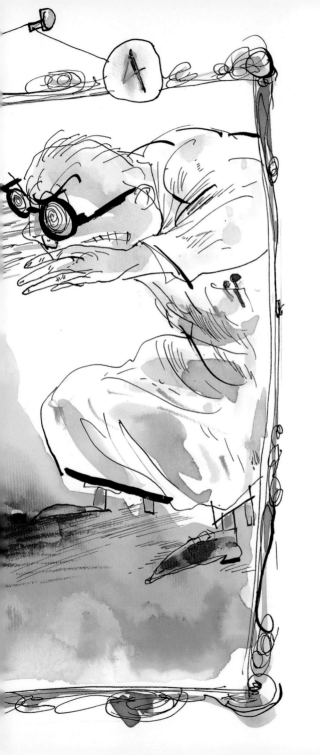

My name is Nico, I can reach your brain in seven seconds

It's Nico for short. In civilian life I'm Nicotine. I'm a dangerous substance, a kind of poison.

When someone loves me and tries to leave me, it takes time. They suffer. I'm a tyrannical bitch, self-centred and highly toxic: I'll do anything to carry on and not be left behind. For me, people get up in the middle of the night. They cross town in pyjamas. They pay a lot. And physiologically too, the high price can often be cancer. I love … I give pleasure to make myself indispensable.

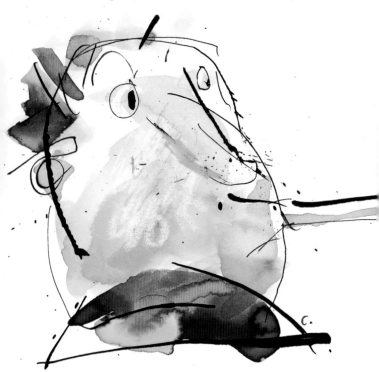

No smoking

I enter by your mouth then, once in your blood,
I penetrate as deeply as possible via the capillaries in
the lungs, as well as via the respiratory and digestive
tracts such as the mouth, the pharynx, the larynx and the
oesophagus. An orgy! It's great! It takes me from seven to
nineteen seconds to reach the brain. There I attach myself
to all kinds of receptors that love me. Called nicotinic
receptors, they are like motorway service stations,
attracting and detaining particular vehicles. Irresistible.
They perceive me, sense me and there I go, on top of
one. They do not see how harmful I am; I hide my true
nature to deceive them. But the results are there to see:
studies have shown that these receptors are increased
by 50 per cent in smokers. When someone loves me …

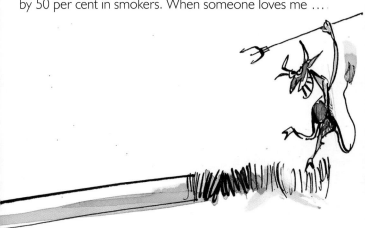

Perseverance.

One smoker in three

tries to stop, but

only one in ten succeeds.

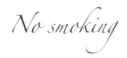

No smoking

Once there, I trigger a sensation of well-being, carried along by a kind of cerebral underground train called dopamine. The result: smokers are hooked because, starting at the brain, I take a stroll through their bodies. And they often ask me why, after two hours, 50 per cent of the Nico they have taken in has disappeared.

'Well hey, the Nico levels have to be restored!' So they have another cigarette, and so on. And what's all this for? To regain the level of Nico that I have artificially raised. This is how the dependence system is created. I make people believe they desperately need me, just as they need to breathe, drink or eat, but it's a completely false impression! With Nico everything's a lie, except for the dependence. I am a fraud who is hard to get rid of. This is the secret of my success, my long life. Got it? Having said this, let's be more retiring and modest: I am just one of some 4,000 substances found in cigarettes. But what harm I do! I constrict the arteries, interfering with oxygenation of the tissues. My unquestioning client's heart uses more oxygen and beats faster than a non-smoker's. I'm a bitch. They know, but they don't care. So I go on. **What luck!**

Help!

95 per cent of attempts to stop

without medical support

end in failure within a year.

No smoking

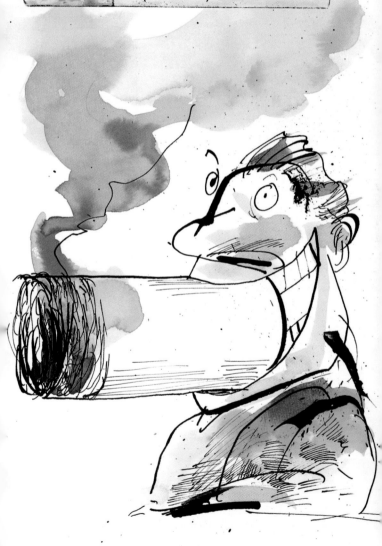

Small world.

There are 1.1 billion smokers

in the world today;

(there will be) 1.7 billion in 2029.

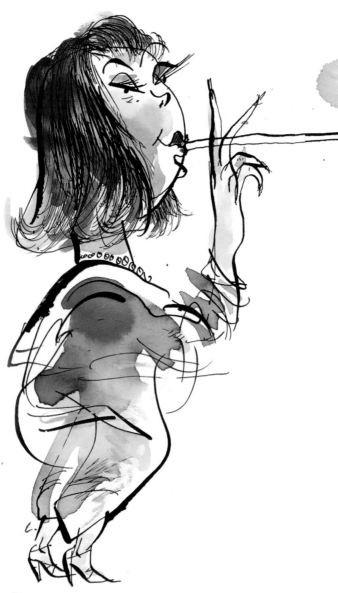

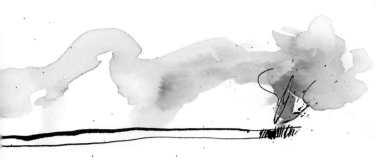

100 days, or three months and a bit later

I stopped smoking 100 days ago. So far I have been successful. Not the tiniest stub since that fateful Tuesday, marked with a red line on my calendar, 'No more fags', finished, forever.

To start with, I didn't believe in the idea. I wasn't sure I'd get there. At the beginning I held on because the decision had been taken, because the patches stuck to my shoulder fed me nicotine, and because the objective was short term (hang on for the morning, start again after lunch, forget the afternoon, make up for it in the evening). It was a daily victory, omnipresent, all-pervading. This didn't prevent irrepressible urges, but I never had to fight the desire to take a cigarette and light it. It's a fine distinction. I have never said to myself: 'Too bad, I'll have one.' To my great amazement I managed to distract myself before getting to that point, every time. Was it because, fairly quickly, I tried to make the thing relative by making this decision a 'non-event?'

No smoking

I don't know. The people around me sometimes noticed that something had changed. The irritability of the ex-smoker cannot be denied either in the office or in the home. If I am to believe the comments, I wasn't insufferable; I was better than predicted. The hardest part was the attack during the sixth week. Non-smoking was beginning to seem normal and it became logical to envisage not smoking any more. I had reached a point where it was useless to think about the time when smoking was pleasant. Support lessened when it was still needed. I suffered. It didn't last long: fifteen days at the most. I took St John's Wort. It passed. Then, bit by bit, I was overcome by a feeling of pride. Well, I'm holding

Example. When both parents smoke, 44 per cent of boys and 37 per cent of girls also smoke. When neither smokes, the figures are 29 per cent and 9 per cent respectively.

No smoking

on. By now smoking seemed futile. Stopping required so much effort that I wouldn't start again for anything in the world. Even if ex-smokers keep on wanting to smoke for some years, I will manage to control these urges. And my weight? I put on 3 kilos (6.6 lb). I'll lose them. I've crossed to the other side. I'm proud of it.

On going back to the office, I discovered that two colleagues had decided to stop as well. With all my heart I wish them every success. And I wish success to those who promise that they will do it soon. You can't know exactly when you will feel better. It's definitely the least describable effect of this endeavour. **But it's the most important.**

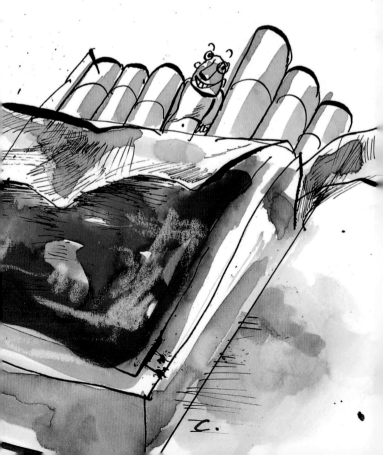

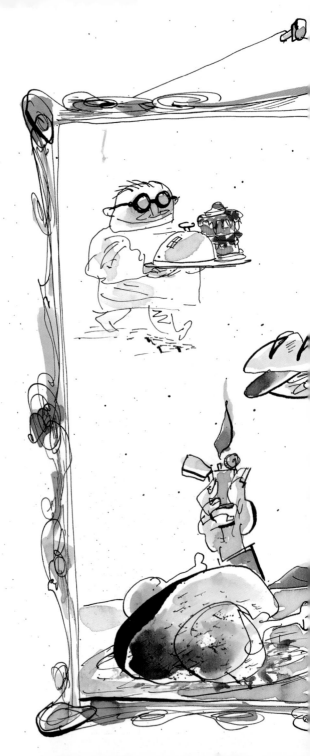

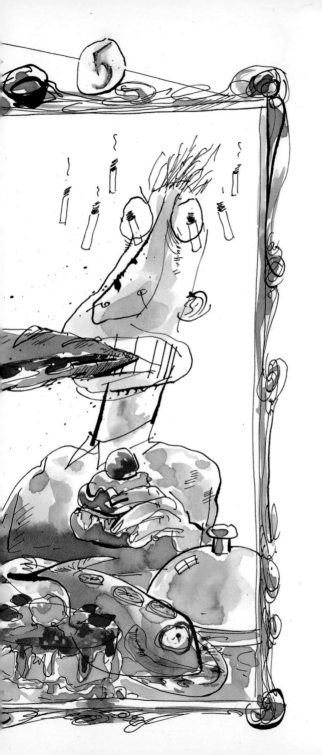

5 kilos (11 lb) gained: managing my wardrobe problem

In the beginning you tell yourself it's not serious. That 'all this will go back to normal' all by itself. Without having to think about it or make any effort. Wine, beer, steak and chips, hamburgers, snacks, nibbles and as much cheese as you like: above all, no change in diet. Don't rely on comments made by others, including your friends, to dispel doubts.

'Hell, I'm getting fat!'
'Not at all!'
'I can't get into my trousers.'
'It's incredible, it doesn't show at all!'

This conversation closely resembles a soft excerpt from *Sex and the City*.

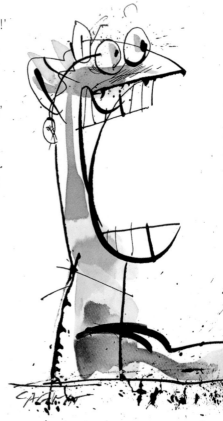

No smoking

You will have to go through it. In such cases, men can become simplistic and cowardly, and look for fake reasons to explain what is obvious. Trousers that are too small have shrunk in the wash, in the dryer (away with these dryers that ruin everything), when being ironed; or there's a serious problem with the cloth or even the cut. It's the container that's at fault, certainly not the contents (you). Then the truth takes over. Some signs are unmistakeable. With yours truly, for example, rolls of fat appear when I'm sitting down, especially at the edge of the bed or on the 'throne'. These are ideal moments for self-appraisal, intimacy is at its height, there's nobody to look or make comments.

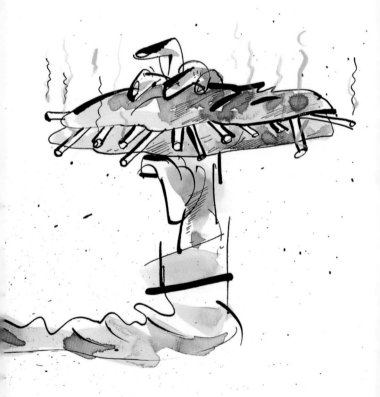

No smoking

Contracting the few abdominal muscles I possess,
I measure the roll(s) of fat on my stomach between
the thumb and index finger of my left hand (I am left-
handed). If all is well, the interval separating them is
not more than two or three centimetres. When I am
overweight, this can triple, with decided sideways
overflow. How awful. Then I repeat the action several
times, but it's difficult to lie to myself. As the length of
time since stopping increases, so also does the
distance between the two digits … By a few
millimetres, yes, but in the end there is a gain of
5 kilos (11 lb). The other sign is on the thighs;
to be precise, the upper thighs. The excess
weight settles there. From
now on, they touch each
other. It's a loathsome
feeling. Together with
the rolls that form
(obviously you can't
have one without
the other), it's a lot.

No smoking

In any case, we are forced to admit that trousers that were 'the right size' when bought, quickly become too short, just a little too short, as soon as a few kilos appear. Not to mention shirt collars, jackets and belts; even my watchstrap had to be let out. Sports car drivers who use a close-fitting safety harness, not an extendable safety belt, know what I'm talking about: the tiniest 'gain' is annoying. Four months after stopping, my assets have increased by a good 5 kilos (11 lb). What should I do? A French Prime Minister (Raymond Barre) and a German Chancellor (Helmut Köhl) had two wardrobes at their disposal for the pre- and post-slimming periods. Not me. Firstly, I have to tell myself that this transient overload is for a good cause. These are good kilos. They were expected, inevitable. Anyway, I'd been told about it.

Doctor G. gave me three months to lose them. And some good advice: stop alcohol completely for a month

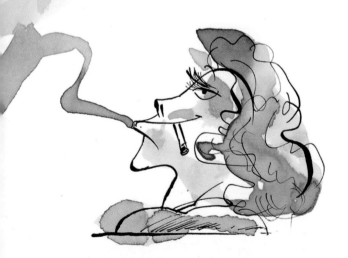

No smoking

and definitely lose 2 kilos (4.4 lb). No more cheese, except at breakfast. Nothing between meals, for pity's sake. Above all, no peanuts, pistachios, hazelnuts and other tasty little things before lunch or dinner – they're fatal! Sport, if possible, at the rate of two sessions a week, and ideally a daily jog. There you are! Easily said. All this, while practising the tiny daily deceptions that show that we are only human. Yes, 'only just' fitting into an article of clothing in the morning can put you in

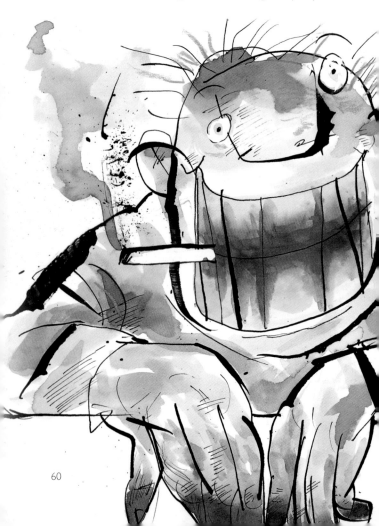

No smoking

a bad mood, or even make you feel sad for the whole day. No, it's not insuperable. Stopping smoking has made me mature and think about the quest for well-being so much that the effort expended on losing a few kilos does not seem inordinate, compared with the battle against tobacco I have just won. I have freed myself from nicotine. I will do the same with these rolls of fat. Stopping smoking amounts to a permanent positive-thinking treatment. It's much more than an isolated action against nicotine. Too bad if I keep these kilos. **My wife said it doesn't worry her ... and I have no mistress.**

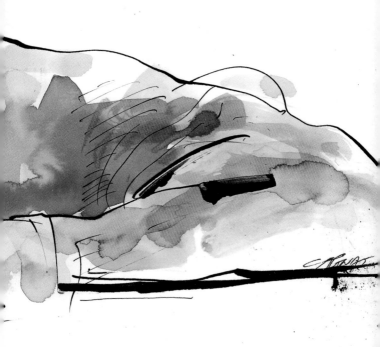

No smoking

The benefits of a
vinicultural weekend:

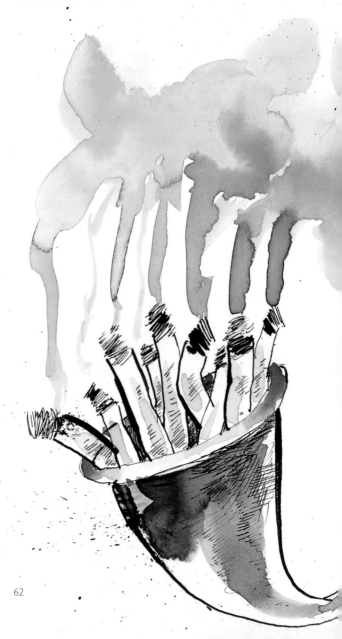

rediscovering taste and the smell of my dearly beloved (MDB)

A friend, a great lover of pipes and cigars, is celebrating his fortieth year in Burgundy, the famous French wine-growing region. It is his wife's idea: she has invited several couples. On the programme is two days" tasting near the town of Beaune. I don't know a great deal about wine. I know how to drink them well enough, and possibly

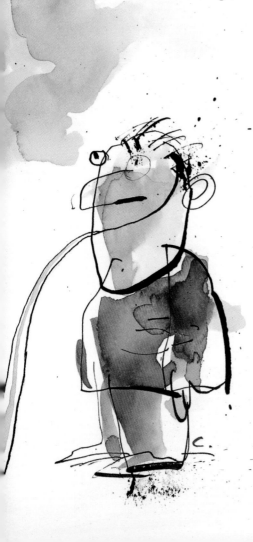

distinguish claret from burgundy (just), but certainly not burgundy from a Loire wine. I have gained great pleasure throughout my life, drinking wine with the family, with my brothers, or in professional situations. I have tasted some great wines, and have appreciated them – obviously not to the extent of their true value. However, they say that oenologists (and other enlightened wine buffs) who are smokers can call on their olfactory memory – which allows them to do their job – despite the effect of cigarettes. I thought I could recognise a good wine. I believed I was endowed with a capacity to recall tastes accurately. But in reality, as regards taste buds and nose, I was a handicapped person.

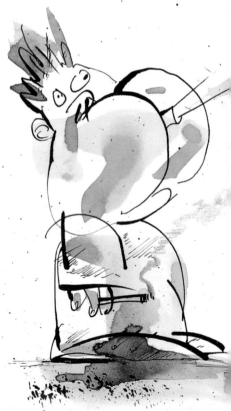

No smoking

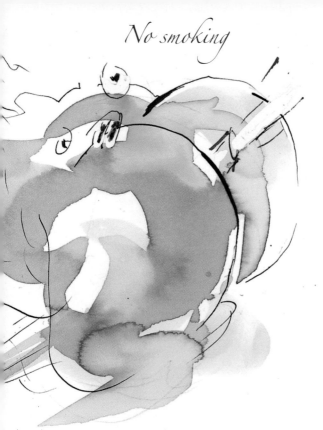

The risk of bladder cancer occurring in smokers is multiplied by 2.5 in men and by 5 in women. This cancer is caused by substances in the smoke that reach the bladder via the blood and are eliminated in the urine, thus spending some hours in contact with the walls of the bladder.

No smoking

Tasting wine in Burgundy meant going down into a cellar. It was pretty hot. The owner's daughter took charge of us. A course in tasting: revolve the glass slowly, use your nose, close your eyes and concentrate solely on the nostrils. Start again. Do as the others do: look at the colour in the light. Use your nose again. Drink. Slurp, slurp. The wine passes from one side of the mouth to the other. A gentle gargle. I swallow. No, no, you don't spit it out. Not today. As the vintages were paraded, I began to taste, to perceive something previously unknown to me. As never before, I managed to capture an aroma, to analyse what I was tasting. The development and structure of the taste became palpable. The technical terms ('and there, the persistence on the palate, can you taste it?') meant something, whereas before they meant nothing. What started out as merely a pleasant sensation attributed to the quality of the wine quickly became a revelation. It was clear enough what we were drinking: on that day it was a good, but not famous burgundy. The explanation for my heightened sensations lies elsewhere.

Something happened there in that cellar. There was a before and an after. I have experienced this once before in my life, only once. I was twelve; we were doing oral composition in French. Until then, I had been a very average student but, for once, I had learned my lesson

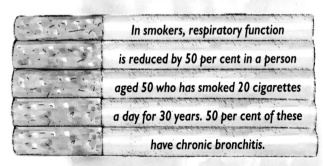

In smokers, respiratory function is reduced by 50 per cent in a person aged 50 who has smoked 20 cigarettes a day for 30 years. 50 per cent of these have chronic bronchitis.

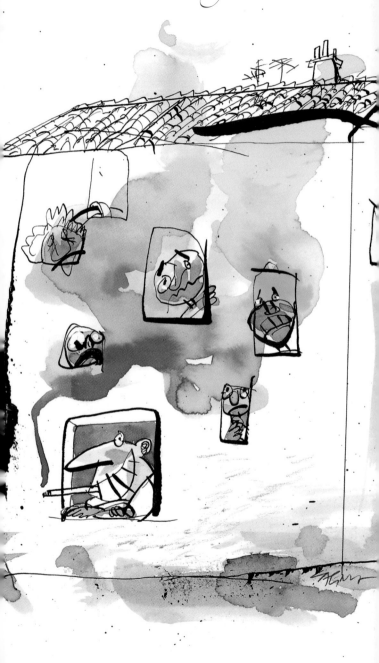

No smoking

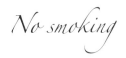

really well. I was listening to a student being examined. As he recited, something clicked inside me. Everything became easy, obvious. A few minutes later when the teacher examined me, he couldn't believe his ears. He was stupefied. I had come good. Congratulations. There you are. And since then I have had no problems with French. The click came again in Burgundy.

I humbly admit to having bent my elbow conscientiously over the last ten years, drinking all kinds of drinks of various qualities. But I was not very discerning. It was as though there had been a plastic film over my palate and nostrils for years, and it was suddenly removed. Incredible, but true. Then I concentrated more on my nose than on the sensations in my mouth to make sure that too much alcohol wasn't the true, serious cause of

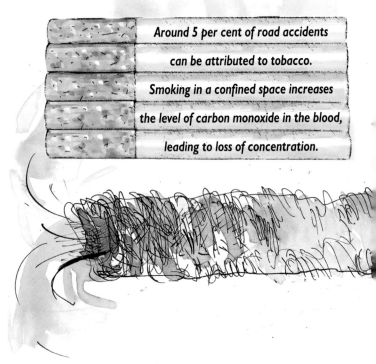

Around 5 per cent of road accidents can be attributed to tobacco. Smoking in a confined space increases the level of carbon monoxide in the blood, leading to loss of concentration.

No smoking

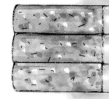

Smoking over 15 cigarettes a day

is the second largest factor,

after the sun, in ageing the skin.

this impression. No. It was verified taking an aperitif, and then again at dinner. The wine breathed as never before. This was a weekend of complete (re)discovery. Wanting to take the process from end to end, I told myself I should try to rediscover as many olfactory experiences as possible. Nothing better than MDB for that. I rest my nose on her neck and close my eyes. I swear, the effect was the same. Forgotten scents return. I smell 'scraps of aroma' (yes, yes) of our children. And not a day passes without my being overwhelmed by this feeling. A detergent, a notebook, a new car … everything is fodder for the olfactory memory. An entire section of my life surfaces again thanks to my nose. Fabulous. Thanks for the weekend. **And the cigarettes can get lost!**

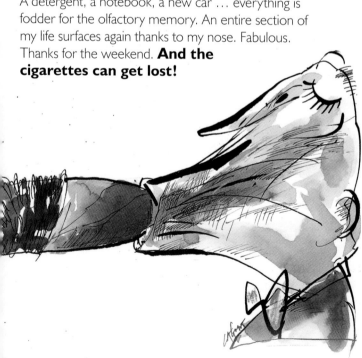

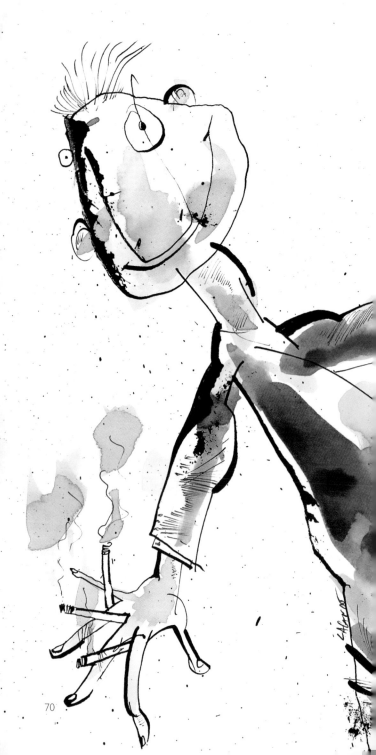

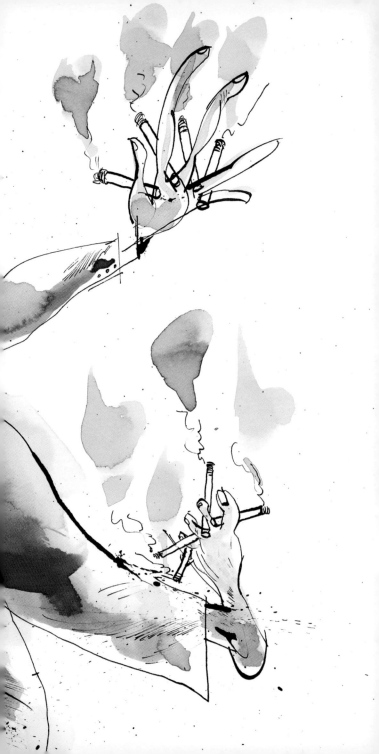

No smoking

I'd like those I love to stop too, or never start

Dear Capucine, Felicity, Viola, Gaspard, Nicolas, Chloë,
Arthur, Jules, Jean, Ella, Josephine, Laetitia, Eugenie,
Louise,
Dear children, nieces and nephews,
Your ages run from one to fourteen years old. You are
the ones I love the most and who should never start
smoking. When I was as old as my eldest, I was already
smoking a cigarette after lunch every day and another
after school – perhaps even two. Strong Virginia or dark
with no filter, depending on what I could find in someone
or other's pockets – packets belonging to my parents or
friends. In the evening, in the absence of cigarettes, I would
borrow one of my father's pipes, timing ten minutes by
my watch, the time it takes to go and put my moped away

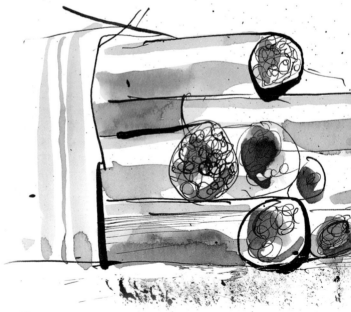

No smoking

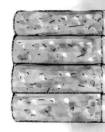

50 per cent of smokers die prematurely because of tobacco. 25 per cent of smokers will not reach the age of retirement.

in the garage and take a few puffs. Sometimes, when the pipe was not properly clean, I had the unpleasant surprise of tasting pure nicotine juice in my mouth. I wasn't even disgusted by it. Appalling, when you think about it. Back in the house, given the state of my breath, it became an absolute priority to avoid the goodnight kiss. When you reach a certain age, you might say that parents check your breath each time you say goodnight. You'd be mistaken!

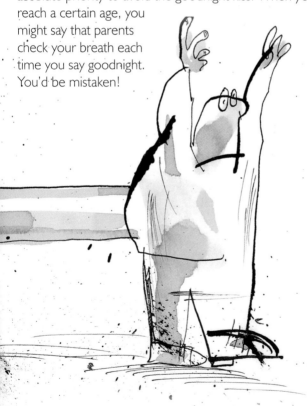

No smoking

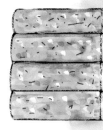

Women in danger. With women smokers on the increase, the incidence of lung cancer in women will overtake that of breast cancer by 2025.

I had started smoking at the age of twelve, sneaking cigarettes in the house, smoking them in haste, and following them up right away with a good dose of chocolate and peppermint chewing-gum. My parents smoked dark cigarettes. My mother stopped smoking when I took it up. I ended up by sneaking more coins than packets of cigarettes … sorry. Then I grew up in a smoker's world. According to the experts, this is a definite handicap.

Is there an infallible method to prevent our children ever trying it? Tobacco manufacturers would pay a huge amount to suppress it if so.

Children, spare yourself (and us) this torture. Smoking is expensive; so expensive it is well worth investing in some other pleasure – something real: a CD, a film, a

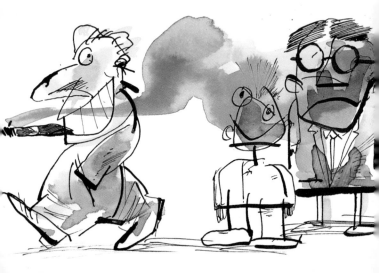

No smoking

pair of jeans, a pair of shoes, a day out. Don't do any favours to cigarettes or to those who manufacture them. Think of them *en bloc* as an adversary, a personal enemy. Have you smoked already? It's disgusting, isn't it? The first puffs inevitably are not very nice. And you haven't even managed to inhale the smoke yet … and you never will (because you won't smoke). Say to yourself that this

	Cancer.
	36 per cent of cancers in men, and
	4 per cent in women are due to tobacco.

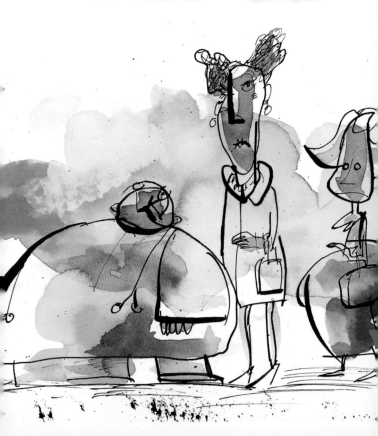

thing, at its worst, is as serious as the other drugs, since in the end it puts you in danger of dying. You are eleven, twelve or fifteen years old? Have you needed cigarettes to revise your homework so far? No. Have you needed cigarettes after lunch or dinner? No. Have you needed them to keep your street cred in front of others? Well, then, you don't need them.

The great difference between me and you is the level of information. In our day, we didn't know everything. Medical knowledge was a long way from what it is today. Since tobacco has become Public Enemy Number 1, you can check how poisonous it is any time you like. Don't let yourselves be influenced as we were. Don't become victims. Don't be weak. Reject manipulation. You are the toughest consumers, the most demanding, the best informed in our society, way ahead of adults …

You know all about a product, brand and style before it wins you over. Do the opposite with smoking. See the evil it causes. Make an investment of will power, perseverance and interest in dealing with it. Life will repay you a hundredfold.

Long. You have to smoke for 30 years on average for most of the effects on health to be detected.

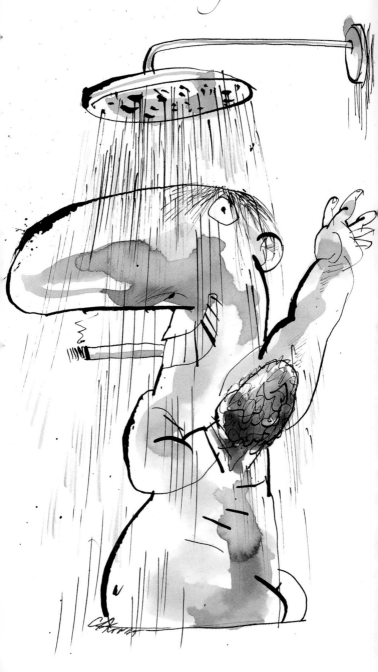

No smoking

There are also those who should stop. They will recognise themselves: around forty, working, damaged by life. One of them is my brother, the third of four. In my family 75 per cent of my siblings smoked. The level fell to 25 per cent in six months: two stopped, not bad. The third brother and his wife still haven't stopped. You can't force them. You just tell them that you care about them and that, given the statistics, there's a fair chance that one of the four will catch 'something'. It takes fifteen years to reduce the risk of lung cancer by 50 per cent. But the good news is that pre-cancerous cells are replaced by healthy cells after about ten years. The sooner you stop, the further the risk recedes. A personal message: if you can use the will power you have already applied to successful projects for the last fifteen years, you have the strength to stop smoking.

What are you waiting for?

Smoking increases the risk of difficulties with erection (increasing equally with age). At 50, the frequency goes from 56 per cent with less than 20 cigarettes a day to 60 per cent with more than that, compared with 27.7 for non-smokers.

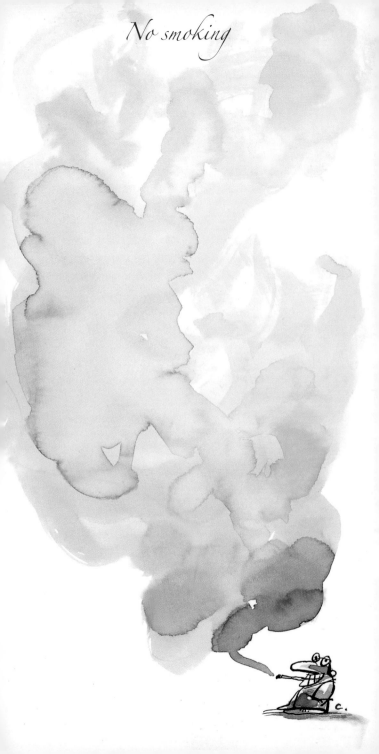
No smoking

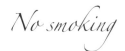

No smoking

What am I gaining? Time, money, other things. How I congratulate myself

Financially the gain is the equivalent of one or two packets a day. With inflation, the sum quickly increases. You can say the money is being put to 'good use'. This first incentive has the great merit that it can be thought of as motivation.

Are cigarettes expensive? Yes. Does stopping smoking allow you to save? No, not at the beginning. Stopping is a pretty burdensome treatment, the price of which has apparently been taken into consideration. A month of patches costs about as much as a month of cigarettes. What rotten luck! The £67 or so that I thought would no longer go up in smoke during the first month took the form of stickers to be applied every day to my arms, my shoulders – a different place every day, if you please. You then pass some weeks dreaming about the cigarettes you have sworn not to smoke: you chuck the tobacco budget into patches and buy yourself presents to forget about it. It is essential to celebrate your progress as often as you need to: the first day, the second, at home, in the office, with your friends, your wife's friends, the friends of your friends. Whoever you want. Any reason will do. First week: a shirt! Second week: a suit! 'A real bargain, darling, you've never seen a sale like it.' By the third week, stopping takes on the nature of a non-event. You add things up … and calm down. You begin to use cold reason. Not smoking means not needing to have money to buy cigarettes; it's avoiding any temptation that might tend to create too much desire.

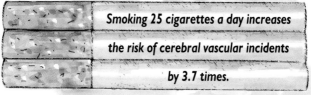

No smoking

Smoking 25 cigarettes a day increases the risk of cerebral vascular incidents by 3.7 times.

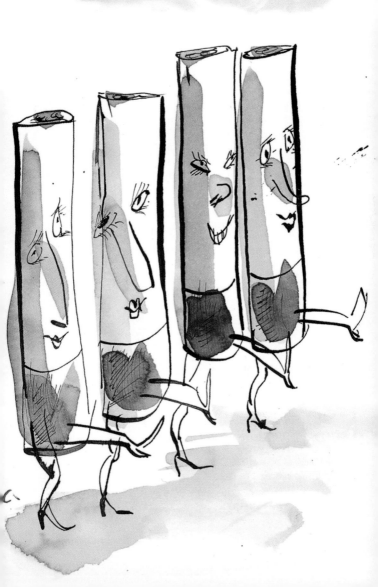

No smoking

I have drastically changed my morning routine. I used to stop for the papers, coffee, and possibly a packet of cigarettes. That's over. Instead I gain some time. I reclaim it as leisure. I buy two or three times fewer tickets from the lottery kiosk than before. Thus, without wanting to, the ex-smoker becomes the miser on duty who never has a penny on him. Any means to an end, and this is another to help me achieve it.

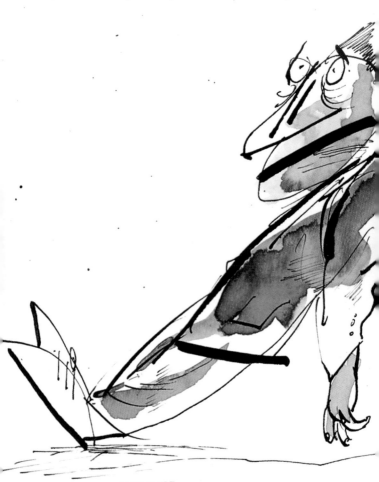

No smoking

The ex-smoker sometimes has a slight predilection for beer or a glass of red wine at the bar. By quitting one dependence and not wanting to be drawn in again right away, he avoids these end-of-the-day diversions. It's a dangerous way of congratulating oneself.

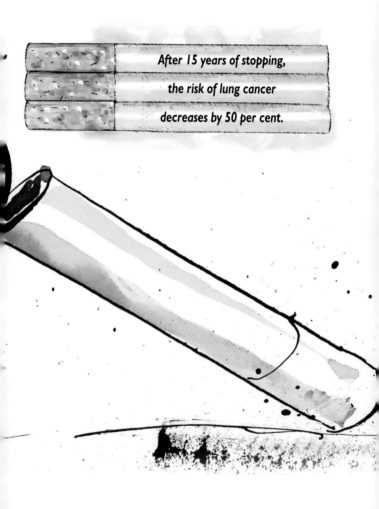

After 15 years of stopping,

the risk of lung cancer

decreases by 50 per cent.

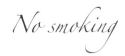

No smoking

'OK, just one and I'm off. They're waiting for me'.
He knows this tune. Before, it was 'One last one,
before I go …' And then very often it was two …
Anyway, the percentage of ex-smokers who become
alcoholics is infinitesimally small.

By the second month I motivate myself by thinking of
the money I've saved. I've stopped the patches, the
smoking kit no longer exists. I have £100 to blow every
month – guaranteed pleasure. I bought myself some golf
lessons. I had taken up this sport some years previously,
but not very seriously. I viewed on starting up again as a
compensation for smoking, a potential source of pleasure.
I will stop smoking but I'll become good at golf. I just had

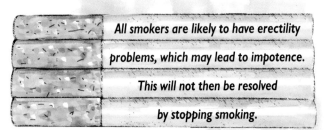

All smokers are likely to have erectility

problems, which may lead to impotence.

This will not then be resolved

by stopping smoking.

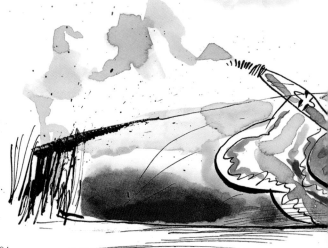

No smoking

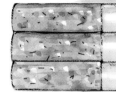

55 per cent of men

who stop smoking put on

at least 3 kilos (6.6 lb).

the wrong sport. Golf is technical, complicated … It calls for such regularity, such application, that having fixed his goals, the golfer becomes an addict; he thinks of nothing else, sometimes to the detriment of basic things such as the family, because for a game of golf you have to free up an entire half day. In fact, the excuse calling for family effort lasts two months.

Well, all that time I wasn't smoking.

'Fine. Thank you. And as an ex-smoker you stop loving it? This non-smoking of yours is an easy excuse.'

Let's not go too far, not smoking any more doesn't mean you can go to excess in other matters. Allowing yourself some fun doesn't mean acting against your nearest and dearest. I have sometimes tended to ignore this fundamental equation, believing that quitting was a privilege permitting any kind of excess. **Not so, there's a limit to everything, even self-congratulation.**

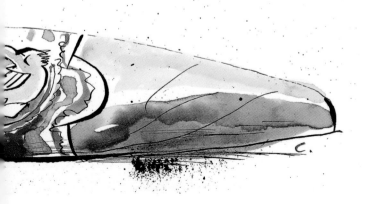

No smoking

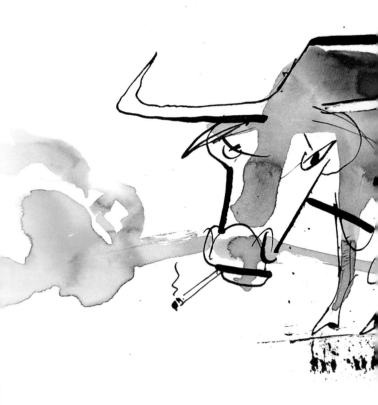

5 years after quitting the risk of

developing cancer of the mouth, throat

or oesophagus will have diminished

by 50 per cent.

No smoking

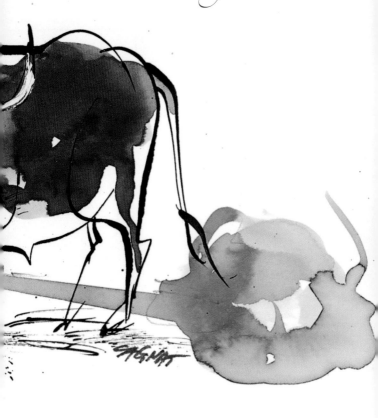

12 years after quitting the risk

of coronary disease becomes

the same as that in a person

who has never smoked.

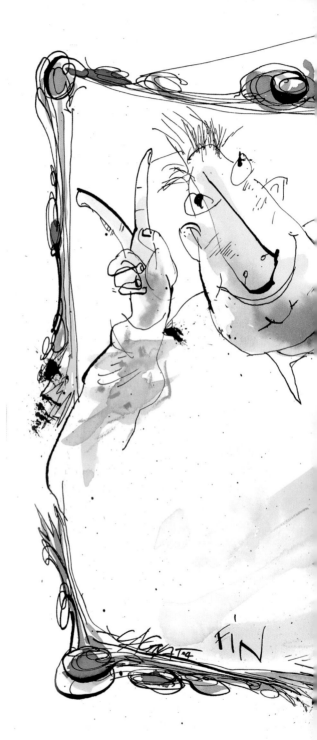

FIN

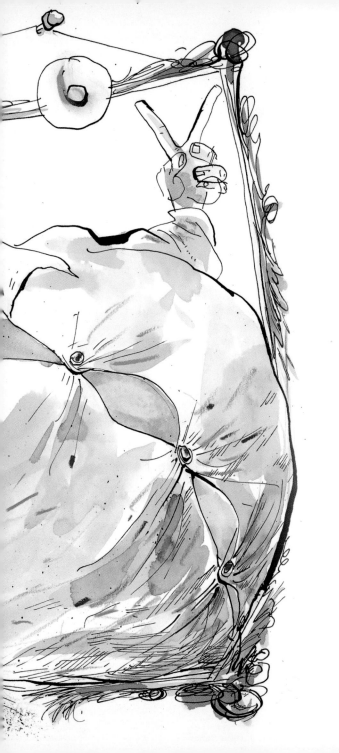

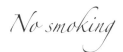

Six months later: free!

A few days after stopping, I told myself I'd start smoking again at seventy-five. That's rich. Each cigarette means living eleven minutes less, the scientists say. At the age of forty the statistic stakes really begin to mean something, all the more so when one has young children. But at seventy-five what do they mean? To take up smoking again in the evening of one's life and suddenly shorten it by three hours each day, what does that change? A month and a half per year: that's nothing. But this is a very bad way to look at things.

In the beginning I was forced to stop. The doctor, my family and society convinced me it was the best thing to do. Deep inside, I remained hooked. I told myself that I would start again some day.

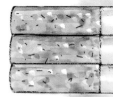

The risk of impotence is multiplied by a factor of 26 in smokers with arterial hypertension.

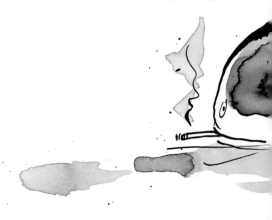

90

No smoking

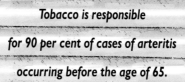

Tobacco is responsible for 90 per cent of cases of arteritis occurring before the age of 65.

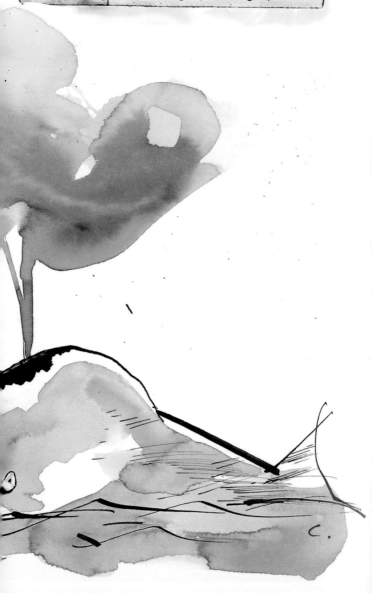

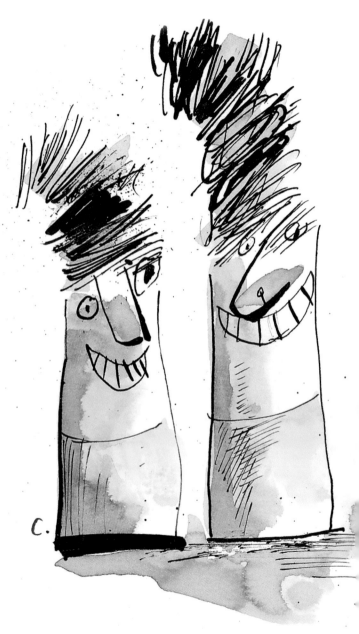

C.

No smoking

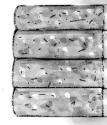

During the 10 minutes approximately it takes to smoke a cigarette, the smoker only inhales smoke for a total of 30 seconds.

Viscerally tied to the moments of pleasure associated with tobacco, I dreamed of it all the time. From getting up to going to bed. Sometimes smoking blanks. I refused to give up what I considered a pleasure, a real one. I regretted the decision many times but I never got near a relapse. I was monitored medically by a doctor, supported by a patch and psychologically prepared, surrounded. I was protected. But I screwed up. Stopping smoking is really a return to normality disguised as D-day. It's a non-event, that's the secret. It's absolutely essential to turn this 'anniversary' into a non-anniversary, to satisfy oneself with nothing, to do without, cheerfully and in good humour. Six months on, frankly I am happy, really happy. Pleased with myself. The score is: Nicotine 0, Pierre (me) 1. I'm glad to have held on, to have managed to draw a definite line under it. This certainty is forged gradually. It first establishes itself because you have to endure such suffering to stop that you don't want to live through it again, too much effort. Go backwards? No. That's the first click.

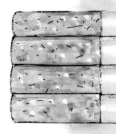

Weight. For every 20 cigarettes per day, the body at rest uses about 250 to 300 extra calories.

No smoking

After that you tell yourself that the feelings acquired as
the weeks pass are worth it: getting up in the morning
without a furry mouth or a headache, even after
an evening drinking and a short night's sleep; being
complimented on your sparkling complexion. As the
days pass, the desire remains, but the reasons for starting
again recede because they become futile. It has taken
six good months for the absence of tobacco to become
a daily pleasure, a real source of joy and pride.
Like a schoolboy with good marks, I surprised myself
counting the weeks and wanting to celebrate the passage
of time. You can't imagine how happy it makes me to
kiss a child, or my wife, without having to hold my
breath discreetly before putting lips to cheek, for fear
of causing displeasure.
All that is finished. Stopping smoking is like repairing an
old house that you have completely fallen in love with,

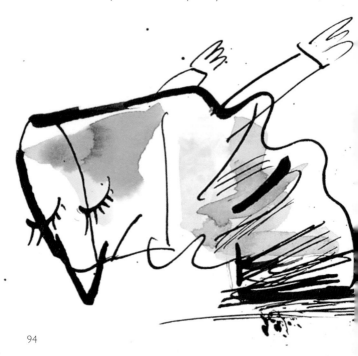

No smoking

and giving it back its early years. It's a new start as well as a renewal. Nicotine yellows the teeth, gives you a grey complexion, blocks your arteries, ruins your lungs, and I'll do without it.

There's a desire to put everything right, bit by bit. Dropping tobacco frees the body and the mind. The palpable sensation of freedom you have is followed by a great desire for natural restoration: you remove the stucco from a dirty façade. It has the same effect. Does the cloud of smoke that accompanies a smoker fuddle his brain as well? Anyway, that's how it happened with me. I am now an ex-lover of cigarettes. I would not assess at what point it lured me, wound me up, abused me and did me harm. I've stopped.

I hope never to suffer from cancer and consequently have to explain to my nearest and dearest why I have it. I hope not to die of it. **That would be too stupid.**

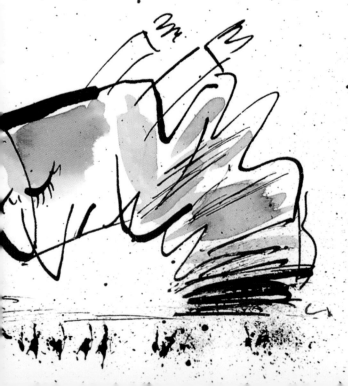

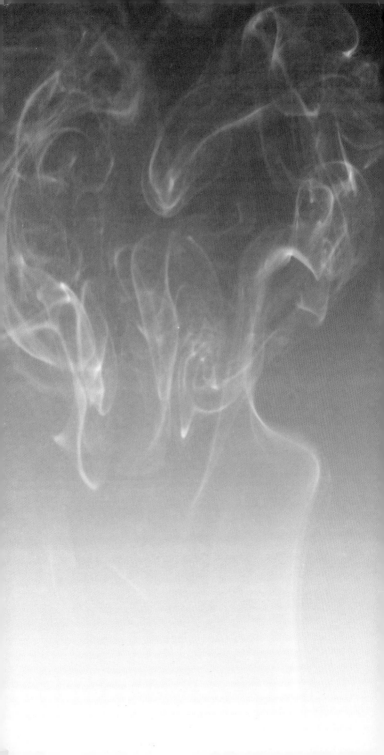